LIVING GOOD

FOR A

FULFILLING LIFE

A 30-Day Daily Guide To Encountering Real Health

Table Of Content

Conclusion.

Introduction

Sarah was a young woman in her mid-thirties who had decided to have a persistent immune system condition that left her feeling tired, in anguish, and struggling to finish even the least difficult of everyday endeavors. Disappointment had seeped into her life as she fought with the limits her health put on her. Sarah came to the medical clinic where I was working then and she scheduled an arrangement and we began.

I had long been something other than a doctor to my patients; I was an assistant, a guide, and an encouraging sign. This particular patient, Sarah Thompson, came into my life and created a lifelong mark on both my career and my point of view on medicine.

From our very first gathering, I moved beyond the standard clinical norms. I spent efforts acquiring not solely Sarah's clinical past however in addition her manner of living, her everyday timetables, and her close-to-home state. I agreed that an individual's general prosperity was unexpectedly tied to their genuine well-being, and I intended to handle all elements of Sarah's existence.

Together, we departed on an expedition of transformation. I advocated a fair eating routine that comprised mitigating dietary types to aid with coping with her issue. I familiarized her with introspection and breathing practices to alleviate pressure, which might trigger eruptions. I encouraged her to engage in mild activity, custom-made to her capabilities, to forestall muscle deterioration and keep up with joint adaptability.

Nonetheless, what placed me away was my accentuation on the "manual for living good daily." I agree that tiny, trustworthy alterations to everyday propensities may accomplish enormous improvements in one's general prosperity. I provided Sarah with a tailored plan that comprised rising simultaneously every day, placing shortly in care, making out realistic targets, and eating the correct feasts

As the weeks changed into months, Sarah started to observe changes. The aggravation was still apparent, nevertheless, it was more reasonable. Her energy levels increased, and she ended up more pulled in with life. The daily appreciation exercise had switched her emphasis from how she was unable to treat what she could, producing an inspiring viewpoint that poured into many elements of her life.

My technique wasn't simply about clinical therapy; it was linked up with motivating Sarah to seize leadership over her life. I instructed her that the body and mentality were interrelated and that preserving both was important for real healing. Through his instruction, Sarah realized the power of taking care of oneself, the relevance of a strong local region, and the flexibility that resides inside every one of us.

The expedition wasn't without problems. There were days when suffering seemed to overshadow progress and minutes when discontent took measures to repair our devoted work. However, I was normally there with encouraging words, telling Sarah that recovering was a cycle, not a target.

Over the long extent, Sarah's narrative circulated throughout the institution, encouraging various patients to take on a similar approach to dealing with their well-being. My effect stretched out a long way beyond clinical schematics; I had changed into a fountain of enthusiasm for confronting life's obstacles with effortlessness and certainty.

Sarah's procedure was not merely an account of a specialist and his patient; it was a demonstration of the amazing power of an integrated strategy to cope with affluence. My guidance had helped Sarah cope with her problem as well as continue with a good existence every day — one filled up with reason, appreciation, and the knowledge that she had the gadgets to battle any barrier that came her direction.

PART 1

Week 1: The Foundation Of Health

The basis of wellness envelops an all-encompassing technique to deal with well-being that goes beyond the basic deficiency of disease. It's a broad-reaching state of being that incorporates physical, mental, close-to-home, and social success. With a focus on proactive and preventative measures, health intends to build a fair and pleasant existence. This thought has developed conspicuousness as individuals attempt to increase their overall personal contentment.

Day 1: Welcome to Your Real Health Excursion

Leaving on a real health experience is an outstanding endeavor that paves the way for an existence of essentialness and flourishing. Inviting oneself to this excursion includes anything other than putting forward health aims; about accepting a complete technique to deal with well-being that integrates your head, body, and soul.

The most crucial element in welcoming oneself to your actual health undertaking is self-acknowledgment. Perceive that this adventure is exciting to you, and your initial stage is right where you should be. There's no need to concentrate on comparing yourself with others, nevertheless about finding out your advantages and locations for improvement. Embrace your imperfections and regard them as any open avenues for advancement.

Then, put forward expectations different than unbending aims. Rather than concentrating simply on weight reduction or real triumphs, contemplate what you need to complete concerning by and large flourishing. Would you wish to grow your energy levels, concentrate on your psychological clearness, or lessen pressure? Adjust objectives to the more wide vision of feeling better and more lively in your day-to-day routine.

Focus on taking care of oneself is a crucial aspect of any true health quest. This involves supporting your body with nutritious dietary choices, maintaining hydrated, and taking part in daily physical work that you like. Recollect that consistency matters more than power. Make tiny, sensible modifications that steadily get coordinated with your way of life. Develop care all through your vacation. Focus on how your body replies to diverse dietary sources, activities, and stresses. Pay heed to your body's indications and alter your methods properly. Integrate habits like introspection or writing to stay linked with your opinions and emotions. Care supports you with settling on mindful selections that help your prosperity.

Encircle oneself with a solid local area. Share your expectations with companions, relatives, or similar persons who can supply support and responsibilities. Having an organization of persons who understand your approach might have a terrific effect on your inspiration and duty. Commend your successes on the way, regardless of how tiny they may look. Each step you take towards a better way of life is a success. Recognize your development and give yourself credit for the excellent adjustments you're making. Recall that your actual wellness venture is a continuing cycle. There's no need to concentrate on reaching out about adopting a deep-seated commitment to your success. Show control toward oneself, and grasp that mistakes are a typical component of the excursion. What is vital is your preparedness to continue pushing forward and consistently take a shot at higher wellness.

In welcoming yourself to your actual health initiative, you're beginning out on a route of self-disclosure, progress, and strengthening. Embrace the cycle, keep open to learning, and let your journey be an imprint of your dedication to live your best, best life.

Day 2: Careful Wake-up Routines: Beginning Your Day Right

Careful wake-up practices are a good approach for starting your day with a goal, inspiration, and a sense of peace. By incorporating cautious practices into your morning routine, you create an inspiring vibe till the finish of the day and build a setup for more noticeable focus, efficiency, and generally speaking success.

1. Awaken Carefully: Start your morning by delicately waking without surging. Rather than instantly running for your telephone or springing up, spend a couple of seconds to become attentive to your ambient elements and the feelings in your body. Take a couple of deep breaths and express appreciation for the new day.

2. Stretch and Move: Take part in gentle stretches to excite your body. This might comprise easy yoga poses, neck and shoulder rolls, or even a brief stroll. Moving your body further promotes blood dispersion and establishes a great genuine tone for the day ahead.

3. Careful Relaxing: Commit a few seconds to focused breathing practices. Practice significant, slow breaths in through your nose and out through your mouth. This quiets your sensory system, minimizes pressure, and supports you with turning out to be more present.

4. Hydration: Begin your day by sipping a glass of water. Hydrating your body night-time of slumber helps kick off your digestion and delivers a rise in vitality. Consider combining your water with lemon for an additional purifying touch.

5. Careful Eating: Assuming you eat, do it cautiously. Relish each bite, concentrate on the tastes and textures, and eat without interruptions. Careful eating increases improved processing and produces an elevating mood for your interaction with food throughout the day.

6. Appreciation Practice: Pause for a minute to examine three things you're glad for. Developing appreciation increases your overall state of mind and point of view, producing an inspired atmosphere for the day. You may scribble things down in a journal or simply contemplate them to you.

7. Perception: Put in nearly little time visualizing your day ahead. Envision yourself passing through your tasks and commitments effortlessly, with attention, and vigor. Envisioning accomplishment modifies your viewpoint and expectations.

8. Insistences: Integrate positive certifications into your daily program. Pick a couple of justifications that affect you and rehash them out loud or in your psyche. Certifications may encourage your self-assurance and aid with creating a good mindset.

9. Computerized Detox: Try not to check your telephone or texts when you arise. Give yourself something like 30 minutes to an hour of tech-leisure time. This protects you from being entangled with outside things before you've received a chance to concentrate on yourself.

10. Careful Preparation: Before diving into your errands, demand a handful of minutes to carefully arrange your day. Focus on your responsibilities, put forward reasonable targets, and allocate time for pauses. Careful organizing forestalls overpower and enhances efficiency.

11. Careful Development: If time allows, engage in a careful development activity, like yoga or judo. These practices link real growth with concentrated consideration, supporting you with commencing your day with centeredness and imperativeness.

Day 3: Supplement Rich Morning Feasts: Empowering Your Body

An extra-rich breakfast is a crucial component of starting your day on the correct foot. Recently meal gives the key fuel and nutrients your body needs to send off your processing, center around cerebral inclination, and stay mindful of by and large success.

Right when you pick a morning dinner that is loaded with nutrients, you're essentially supplying your body with the instruments it expects to operate optimally over the day. Supplement-rich food choices are normally ones that are plentiful in supplements, minerals, fiber, and protein while being relatively low in added sugars and bad fats. Coordinating these food components into your morning meal might create the environment for a helpful and optimistic day.

Starting your day with a solid source of protein is vital. Protein modifies glucose levels, manages hunger, and aids muscle maintenance and growth. Eggs, Greek yogurt, curds, and lean meats are outstanding wellsprings of protein that can be effectively incorporated into your morning feast. Whole grains are one more necessary ingredient of an enhancement-rich feast. They give complex carbohydrates that release energy slowly, assuring you feel full and energized for extended intervals. Choose whole grain cereals, oats, whole wheat bread, or quinoa to acquire the benefits of upheld energy release.

Coordinating distinct outcomes of the earth into your morning dinner may aid in its enhanced content fully. These dietary sources are numerous in vitamins, minerals, and disease anticipation experts that increase safe capability and all-around wellness. Consider adding berries, bananas, spinach, or ringer peppers to your morning ritual. Sound fats are equally needed. They assist in captivating fat-dissolvable supplements and give persistent imperativeness. Food assortments like avocados, nuts, seeds, and typical nut spread are great wellsprings of sound fats that can be examined for your morning feast.

Avoiding substantially taken care of and sugary breakfast decisions is crucial. These may accelerate energy blunders and demands later in the day. Pick total, irrelevantly took care of food supplies at whatever point the circumstances permit.

Day 4: Ordinary Hydration Affinities: Water for Significance

Ordinary hydration penchants are a basis for keeping conscious of centrality and by and large success. Water isn't just basic for fundamental significant systems however likewise plays a crucial part in preserving your energy pushes ahead, producing sound skin, promoting retention, and supporting cerebral ability. Creating amazing hydration penchants might greatly contribute to your overall noteworthiness.

To ensure you're keeping appropriately hydrated, making drinking water an expected part of your typical routine is vital. Start your day by sipping a glass of water as you emerge. This helps send off your absorption, wash away toxins that have formed for now, and rehydrate your body evening time of rest. You may add a squeeze of lemon for an extra rise in hydration and a minor piece of L-ascorbic corrosive. Throughout the day, aim to spread your water induction similarly. Pass a reusable water bottle with you to make it useful to taste water all through the day. Set refreshes on your phone or utilize applications that screen your water admittance to aid you with keeping up with consistency all through your hydration points.

Focus on your body's messages. Thirst is an apparent adverse effect that your body needs more water. Make an effort not to overlook it; everything else is comparable, and respond quickly by drinking water. Additionally, concentrate on the color of your urine. Light yellow urine is a symptom of proper hydration, whereas dull yellow or dazzling pee might imply drying out.

Coordinating water-rich food items into your eating routine may also contribute to your hydration goals. Food kinds generated beginning from the earliest stage watermelon, cucumber, oranges, and lettuce have enormous water content and may aid with boosting your fluid entrance.

While water is astounding and the most common strategy for remaining hydrated, other benefits like regular teas and infused water may likewise offer to

Day 5: Moving with Reason: Finding Day to day Active labor

Moving with reason involves engaging in day-to-day genuine employment that lines up with your goals and beliefs, adding not solely to your actual success but also to your general experience of contentment. By putting reason into your growth agenda, you may turn practice from a simple errand into a serious task.

Finding daily genuine employment that resounds with your drive begins with contemplation. Think about what makes the most difference to you. Is it focusing on your wellness, engaging with nature, or establishing a good example for your friends and family? When you differentiate your motivation, you may match your workouts to synchronize. For example, if encouraging a solid way of life is your motivation, you may combine a mix of cardiovascular activities, strength preparation, and adaptability exercises into your regular practice. Every meeting then turns into a step towards your drawn-out wellness targets, putting out the perspiration and effort extra essential. Finding an explanation for growth also requires exploring diverse workouts. You might notice that you like energetic strolls around the park, yoga sessions that center your thoughts, or even high-energy dancing workouts that provide delight. The trick is to try different things with varied workouts until you discover the ones that influence you.

Also, adding reason to your proactive responsibilities might reach beyond private benefits. Participating in cause strolls, participating in local area wellbeing events, or joining bunches that line up with your characteristics may implant your workouts with a higher sensation of significance. In addition to the fact that you are moving for yourself, but at the same time you're contributing to issues you care about. It's crucial to spell up distinct goals that reflect your drive. Rather than merely aiming to run a given distance, think about the objective behind it. Is it true that you are racing to bring concerns to light for a purpose? Could it be considered that you are stimulating yourself to fight specific obstructions? By describing your goals within your motivation, you build a more substantial connection with your activities.

Consistency is crucial when advancing with reason. Treat your active labor as a pledge to yourself and your yearnings. Plan a plan that matches precisely with your usual daily practice. This constancy strengthens the relationship between your motivation and your progress, making it a crucial aspect of your life. Recollect that progress isn't straight 100% of the time. There will be days when inspiration melts away, and errors arise. During such moments, reconnect with your motivation. Remind yourself why you started and how each phase contributes to your overall approach. This viewpoint can reignite your assurance and keep you on target.

Integrating care into your growth might expand your perception of direction. Focus on how your body feels throughout exercising. Notice the increases in your solidarity and persistence. Praise the successes, whether they are genuine accomplishments or great forward leaps.

Moving with design is surely not a one-size-fits-all technique. It's connected with tailoring your proactive chores to your interests, values, and yearnings. Whether you're climbing in nature, rehearsing combative skills, or training for a long-distance race, imbuing reason into your growth may transform your workout daily plan into a pleasurable and controllable practice that enhances both your physical and mental prosperity.

The Day 6: Night Wind-Down: Focusing on Relaxing Rest

Making a convincing night wind-down routine is crucial for concentrating on tranquil slumber and enhancing generally speaking well-being. As the day draws to a conclusion, finding a method meaningful approach to relax and set up your brain and body for rest may greatly enhance the character of your rest and contribute to your overall wellness.

Planning up a continuous rest strategy is crucial. Hitting the sack and rising concurrently constantly controls your body's interior clock, making it easier to drift asleep and arise properly. Consistency sets up your body's regular rest-waking cycle, known as the circadian cadence, which assumes an essential function in improving healthy rest. Lessening receptivity to devices before sleep time is one more important feature of a breezy down everyday timetable. The blue light discharged by mobile phones, tablets, and PCs may suppress the creation of melatonin, a hormone that directs slumber. Consider putting a "screen time limitation" one hour previous to bed to let your cerebrum loosen up and flag that now is the correct time to rest. Taking part in quieting activities may aid in communicating to your body that now is the best moment to calm down. Perusing a book, rehearsing delicate extending or yoga, or washing up may all enhance unwinding. These exercises may bring down emotions of worry and assist the journey from the demands of the day to a more serene outlook.

Care rehearses, like mindfulness or thorough breathing exercises, are fantastic methods for calming down at night. These techniques aid with relaxing the brain, lessen anxiousness, and set you up for a restful night's relaxation. By zeroing focus on your breath or being accessible at the moment, you may abandon the day's issues and generate a psychological space for relaxing.

It is equally vital to Establish a pleasing rest environment. Keep your room chilly, dark, and tranquil. Put resources into a consistent sleeping cushion and pads that suit your solace inclinations. Clean up your area and remove any disturbances that might slow down your relaxation.

Restricting hefty feasts, caffeine, and booze close sleep time might prevent disturbances to your slumber. These drugs may delay processing and impair your body's potential to go into a deep rest cycle. Decide on a small, nourishing snack on the off chance that you're famished before rest. Recording your contemplations or developing a plan for the day for the next day will lessen pressure and cleanse your head. At the point when you put your contemplations on paper, you're less tempted to obsess over them throughout the evening, letting you rest all the more quietly.

Consider developing a sleep time tradition that you like. It might entail trying some sans-caffeine tea, paying attention to relaxing, and practicing gratitude by pondering the wonderful portions of your day. These practices might become ameliorating indications that now is the proper moment to loosen up and move into rest mode. Focusing on a night wind-down regimen is an interest in your success. By finding a method intentional approach to relax, detach from devices, participate in quieting activities, and generate an acceptable rest atmosphere, you're creating a way for soothing and rejuvenating slumber. Recollect that creating a trustworthy wind-down routine takes time, so show discipline toward oneself as you make alterations and locate what comes out greatest for your fresh requirements.

Day 7: Supporting Associations: Developing Significant Connections

Supporting relationships and building strong connections is the basis of a fulfilling existence. These ties provide us with fundamental encouragement as well as contribute to our overall prosperity, pleasure, and self-improvement. Whether they are with relatives, friends, or better halves, vital affiliations need effort, realness, and a certifiable eagerness to put resources into the existence of others.

At the basis of building substantial relationships lies the specialty of undivided attention. While taking part in talks, focus on the speaker, put aside distractions, and hear what they're talking about. By showing that you value their contemplations and feelings, you build a place of refuge where straightforward communication may flourish and understanding enhanced. Come at the matter from the other individual's viewpoint, realize their sentiments, and approve their contacts. This creates a more fundamental sense of trust and a more grounded tie, enabling the relationship to expand beyond superficial cooperation. Put time and energy into spending valuable minutes together. In our rapid environment, it's not straightforward to get preoccupied with our own lives. Notwithstanding, putting forth a knowledgeable endeavor to invest energy with friends and family, engage in joint activities, and develop memories together establishes your connection and enhances your relationship's foundation.

Celebrate both the great victories and the minor wins in one another's life. Whether it's a progress job or accomplishing a specified aim, acknowledging and sharing in one another's successes cultivates a spirit of shared aid and support.

Genuineness is important in building substantial relationships. Be transparent about your opinions, feelings, and ambitions. While it's vital to be considerate, keeping up with straightforwardness preserves a strategic distance from misunderstandings and fortifies the trust between you and the other person. Absolution is another aspect of sustaining connections. No relationship is immune to conflicts or misunderstandings. Figuring out how to forgive and push forward displays your commitment to the partnership and exhibits that you value the association more than grasping emotions of spite.

Regard each other's bounds. Perceive that everyone has their cutoff thresholds and needs for distinct space. Regarding these bounds demonstrates your concern for the other individual's consolation and freedom. Consistently convey gratitude and admiration. Expressing your thanks for having someone in your life and appreciating the beneficial influence they have is a great way to preserve relationships. It reinforces the value you set on the connection and builds up your duty to it.

Adaptability and flexibility are crucial in building durable relationships. Individuals evolve and alter after some time, and relationships should progress close to them.

Embrace change, impart straightforwardly about your demands and goals, and adapt to the motions that happen ordinarily in connections.

Week 2: Wholesome Concordance

Wholesome concordance refers to the fair and synergistic connection between various supplements in our eating regimen that contribute to optimal well-being and flourishing. Accomplishing dietary congruity requires eating diverse food sources that supply basic nutrients, minerals, macronutrients, and micronutrients to the proper extent. This viewpoint highlights that no one supplement can operate in segregation; they all link and sustain each other to keep up with basic physical processes.

In a fair eating routine, macronutrients including carbs, proteins, and fats collaborate to supply energy, construct and repair tissues, and direct metabolic cycles. Carbs deliver rapid energy, whereas proteins supply amino acids required for cell repair and growth. Fats assume a role in chemical production and the preservation of fat-dissolvable nutrients. Micronutrients, like nutrients and minerals, are equally required for dietary congruity. These supplements don't supply energy themselves, nevertheless, they go about as cofactors in distinct metabolic reactions. For instance, vitamin D is vital for calcium intake, which is necessary for bone wellness. Nutrients like A, C, and E are cancer-prevention agents that safeguard cells from injury. Minerals like iron and zinc are crucial for resistive capabilities and digestion.

The notion of nourishment amicability also reaches out to the prospect of food cooperation, where particular food types, when taken together, enhance the retention and viability of supplements. For example, consuming L-ascorbic acid-rich food varieties near iron-rich food varieties may operate on iron absorption. This includes the relevance of individual supplement use as well as the mix of meal variety in a feast.

Present-day counts of calories commonly trend towards handled and accommodation food types, which might disrupt dietary amicability. These food sources may be rich in one supplement but ailing in others, prompting a problematic nature. To achieve dietary congruity, it's critical to concentrate on complete, supplement-dense food kinds like natural items, veggies, entire grains, lean proteins, and sound fats. Customized sustenance likewise plays a role in reaching healthy harmony. Every individual's healthful requirements are distinct given aspects like age, orientation, activity level, and fundamental medical problems. Fitting dietary options to individual demands may ensure that the proper supplements are delivered in optimal quantities.

Day 8: Adjusted Dinners: Making Healthy Snacks

Creating adjusted and nutritious snacks is a crucial component of preserving a solid eating routine and improving by and large prosperity. A sensible lunch delivers the vital nutrients to nourish your body and sustain energy levels throughout the remainder of the day. By completing a selection of nutrition courses, you may cook a supper that delights your taste senses as well as supports your nutritional needs.

A fair lunch generally comprises a variety of macronutrients, particularly carbohydrates, proteins, and fats. Carbs operate as the main source of energy and may be derived from whole grains like earthy-colored rice, quinoa, or entire wheat bread. These complex starches release energy gradually, forestalling abrupt spikes and collapse in glucose levels.

Proteins are important for mending and constructing tissues, and they contribute to a feeling of completeness. Lean protein options like grilled chicken, tofu, beans, lentils, or fish may be included in your meal. Protein preserves muscle wellness as well as assists in the manufacture of chemicals and chemicals. Sound fats, like those tracked down in avocados, nuts, seeds, and olive oil, are vital for cell capacity and the preservation of fat-dissolvable nutrients. Remembering a tiny portion of these fats for your lunch may contribute to satiety and offer a sensation of contentment. Vegetables and organic goods are rich in nutrients, minerals, cancer-prevention agents, and dietary fiber. They add tone, surface, and taste to your meal while delivering different medicinal benefits. Mixed greens, hot peppers, carrots, cucumbers, and berries are fantastic selections to consider. Fiber improves absorption and maintains normal glucose levels.

Making a good lunch also requires being mindful of portion estimations. Overburdening your plate might drive abundant calorie admittance, whereas division control sustains the weight of the executives and forestalls indulgence. Integrating full food types and reducing handled fixings further boosts the nutritional benefit of your supper.

Food selection is one more crucial feature of a fantastic lunch. Eating a varied scope of food sources assures that you acquire a variety of supplements. Trying different things with various fixings and recipes will keep your meals exciting and prevent monotony.

Arranging and preparedness assume a key position in dependably receiving a charge out of adjusted snacks. Feast planning throughout the end of the week or the preceding night might save time during busy mornings. Having several pre-cut veggies, cooked cereals, and protein sources instantly available makes it easier to create a fair meal in a hurry. The aim of producing healthy snacks is to maintain your body with a variety of supplements that support your overall well-being and essentialness. By attentively picking a combination of carbohydrates, proteins, fats, veggies, and organic items, you can ensure that your lunch is both gratifying and healthfully beneficial. Creating adjusted eating a tendency might damage your prosperity over the long term.

Day 9: Careful Eating: Appreciating Each mouthful

Careful eating is a training that challenges us to dial back, be accessible, and truly draw in with our food. In our modern society when feasts are in many ways hurried and distracted, mindful eating encourages us to savor each mouthful, creating a more meaningful link with our body, our food, and the experience of eating itself.

At its heart, cautious eating is bound together with increasing awareness. It entails attention to the tones, textures, tastes, and scents of the meal before us. This elevated attentiveness enhances the physical joy of eating as well as aids us in recognizing and responding to our body's indicators of desire and fulfillment. Enjoying each nibble entails linking every one of the faculties. Before tasting, stop for a minute to observe the visual attractiveness of your meal. Notice its lively variety and the manner it's presented on the dish. As you take that initial bite, focus on the surface as it contacts your teeth and tongue. Is it crispy, silky, or delicate?

The tastes that dance on your sense of taste need to be welcomed and appreciated, whether they're sweet, spicy, bitter, or disagreeable. Biting gently and thoroughly is a fundamental aspect of mindful eating. By chewing each mouthful effectively, you let your body metabolize food all the more efficiently, and you become more responsive to the symptoms of fullness. Biting deliberately drags out the enjoyment of the meal and might prevent gorging since it demands investment for the cerebrum to enlist completeness. Careful eating also invites us to draw in with the close-to-home components of our connection with food. Frequently, we resort to nourishment for consolation, stress relief, or celebration. By being accessible and conscious when eating, we may more quickly grasp our close-to-home triggers and responses to food.

This attentiveness may encourage more careful and better judgments over the long run.

To practice mindful eating, minimizing distractions is crucial. Switch off the television, put aside your telephone, and produce a tranquil atmosphere that lets you concentrate completely on your supper. Thus, you may immerse yourself in the demonstration of eating and fully respect the nourishment you're offering to your body. Developing a cautious eating habit provides many rewards for both bodily and mental success. It may help with weight the executives by advancing improved piece control and lowering indiscreet eating. Careful eating likewise encourages a healthier connection with food, which may help to further develop self-perception and lowered sentiments of guilt or shame surrounding eating.

In a more comprehensive environment, careful eating lines up with care all in all — a training that promotes life right now with aim and non-judgment. Applying attention to eating may pour over into many facets of life, fostering a more attentive and thankful manner to interact with daily encounters.

Day 10: Brilliant Nibbling: Empowering Your Evenings

Brilliant nibbling is a key component in maintaining steady energy levels throughout the day, especially during those afternoon droops when inspiration and center will normally wind down. These minutes often lead to disastrous food judgments, for example, going for sweet or deeply handled nibbles that deliver a quick spike of energy followed by an inevitable disaster. In any event, by taking on a cautious manner to deal with eating and selecting supplement-heavy selections, you may effectively empower your nights without damaging your well-being.

While choosing snacks, it's important to select those that accumulate protein, excellent fats, and complex carbohydrates. Protein and solid fats contribute to satiety, supporting you with feeling fuller for longer, while complex carbohydrates supply a steady arrival of energy. Nuts and seeds are superb options since they include a combination of these components. Almonds, for example, contribute protein and good fats, while full-grain saltines or a tiny bit of natural cereal offer complex carbohydrates.

Another way is to add fiber-rich dietary sources into your nibbles. Fiber aids processing as well as regulates glucose levels, forestalling rapid spikes and dips in energy. Vegetables like carrot sticks or celery with hummus, or a tiny portion of full natural product, are uncomplicated and gratifying selections that contribute to outstanding snacking. Greek yogurt is a versatile nibble that merges protein with probiotics, boosting both energy and digestive wellness. You may boost its healthful value by adding berries, chia seeds, or a sprinkling of honey for a little of pleasantness. Hydration likewise assumes a position in keeping up with energy levels. Here and there, what our bodies read as yearning is thirst. Drinking water or herbal tea near your bites might aid with keeping you adequately hydrated and control unnecessary brushing.

Arranging and planning are crucial components of successful clever eating. By having pre-parceled foods quickly accessible, you're more averse to yielding to the enchantment of candy machines or unpleasant driving selections. Also, skimming names may guide you toward lower-sugar, lower-sodium options, it are more feeding to ensure your bites. Eating a tiny nibble around a little while before your energy usually plunges in the early evening may aid with forestalling the downturn by and large. This proactive practice assures your body has a steady stockpile of supplements to draw from as you push through the chores that need to be done.

Day 11: Investigating Superfoods: Upgrading Your Eating Routine

Superfoods have stood out recently for their power to enhance fewer calories and advance generally speaking well-being. These supplement-rich food sources are typically loaded with essential nutrients, minerals, cell reinforcements, and other profitable combinations that give a variety of medicinal benefits. Integrating superfoods into one's dietary routine may be a persuasive strategy for promoting a healthy way of life.

One of the greatest superfoods is blueberries. These small, energetic berries are noted for their high cancer-prevention agent content, notably anthocyanins, which give them their recognizable variety. Cell reinforcements assume a key function in eradicating damaging free revolutionaries in the body, perhaps reducing the chance of persistent diseases like cardiovascular illness, malignant development, and neurological issues. Another generally considered superfood is kale. This emerald green is a nutritious force to be reckoned with, loaded with minerals A, C, and K, as well as calcium and fiber. Its adaptability enables it to be employed in plates of mixed greens, smoothies, or even as a hard bite when cooked. Kale's supplement thickness makes it an amazing choice for expanding bone wellness, resistant capacity, and solid absorption. Quinoa, sometimes referred to as a "complete protein," is another superfood that has garnered popularity. Dissimilar to other plant-based food choices, quinoa includes every one of the nine essential amino acids, making it a terrific alternative for vegetable lovers and vegetarians wanting to satisfy their protein demands. Moreover, quinoa is rich in fiber, magnesium, and various minerals, contributing to further improved satiety and stopping stomach stomach-associated turmeric, a spice usually used in Indian cooking, has been identified for its calming and cell reinforcement abilities. Curcumin, the energetic ingredient in turmeric, is recognized to assume a position in reducing irritation and perhaps lightening the adverse effects of diseases like joint discomfort. Integrating turmeric into foods or beverages might be a great approach for bridging its potential medicinal benefits. Chia seeds have likewise tracked down their spot among superfoods because of their fantastic nutritious feature. These microscopic seeds are abundant in fiber, omega-3 unsaturated fats, and various minerals. When splattered, chia seeds promote a gel-like surface that may be employed to generate scrumptious puddings or incorporated into smoothies for an increase in vitamins and vitality.

The benefits of superfoods reach beyond physical wellness; they may also support cerebral capacity. Greasy seafood, like salmon, is rich in omega-3 unsaturated fats, which are vital for cerebrum wellness. Omega-3s are recognized to add to further developed memory and attention, making them a vital alternative to any eating routine.

It means a lot to take notice that although superfoods might give different wellness advantages, they are ideal when part of a balanced and varied diet. Depending completely on a few superfoods may cause nourishing uneven characteristics. All things being equal, combining a large number of supplement-heavy food sources assures that all nourishing needs are satisfied.

Day 12: Cooking at Home: Embracing Culinary Imagination

Cooking at home gives substance to culinary inventiveness, letting folks explore new paths regarding tastes, fixings, and ways to generate meals that are delightful as well as aware of their preferences. Embracing this inventive component of cooking may be immensely satisfying, motivating a deeper link with food and an increased sensation of success.

One of the benefits of cooking at home is the possibility to research a great many fixings. From vivid tastes to privately procured food, the kitchen transforms into a jungle gym for trial and error. People may draw encouragement from diverse delicacies all across the earth, imbuing their dishes with particular combinations of tastes that excite the sense of taste. Thus, cooking at home turns into an experience that soars beyond the usual.

Moreover, home cooking considers personalization. With an expanding understanding of dietary preferences and constraints, many individuals hunt down comfort in putting up their meals. Cooking at home encourages folks to adjust foods to meet their dietary needs, whether it is creating without gluten, vegetable lover, or low-sodium alternatives. This degree of control cultivates a deeper link with what we eat, promoting by and large health and satisfaction. Culinary innovativeness stretches out beyond taste to display. Plating a finely produced food may be a wonderful art in itself, demonstrating the attention and work that went into its preparation. From organizing bright garnishes to adorning with unique spices, each dish turns into a smaller-than-average show-stopper. This visual attraction offers an additional element of contentment and could lead typical feasts to seem like an uncommon occasion.

Cooking at home equally cultivates a sensation of success. As individuals organize feasts without any planning, they observe their attempts convert into feeding food. This large outcome might promote clarity and confidence, especially for individuals who are fresh to the culinary industry. There's an enormous pride that accompanies offering a food that was thought, developed, and made wholly by one's own hands. Family and societal relationships may be fostered via home cooking as well. Gathering friends and family around the supper table to have custom-crafted food lays out the doors for critical talks and valuable time together. Cooking for loved ones enables individuals to share their affection and inventiveness, making a lasting effect via the joy of wonderful cuisine.

Also, the presentation of cooking at home may be a thoughtful and stress-easing exercise. Drawing in with fixings, following instructions, and zeroing in on the cooking system may be a sort of care. It provides an opportunity to disengage from the rest of the world and submerge oneself in a concrete experience that unites every one of the senses — sight, smell, taste, touch, and, shockingly, sound. In the contemporary rapid environment, the specialty of cooking at home is at risk of being overwhelmed by the accommodation of takeaway and inexpensive cuisine. Be that as it may, by embracing culinary innovativeness and esteeming the technique associated with organizing meals, folks might rediscover the pleasures of home cooking. It's not just about food; it's about the research, articulation, and linkage that food can bring to our lives. Whether it's an easy weekday meal or a complex end-of-the-week feast, cooking at home gives a place where creative ideas and tastebuds may happily entwine.

Day 13: End of the week Dinner Prep: Getting In an excellent position

End-of-the-week supper prep is a vital technique to cope with establishing yourself in a good position over time. By allocating a period around the end of the week to create, get ready, and portion your meals, you may save time, lessen pressure, and decide on healthier eating options. This training encourages you to assume command over your eating regimen and ensures that you have healthy options quickly accessible, even on the most active of days.

The most crucial aspect at the end of the week supper planning is organizing. Pause for a minute to analyze your upcoming week's schedule. Think about your job duties, plans, and any friendly workouts that may impact your meals. In light of this data, plan out what you'll consume for breakfast, lunch, dinner, and snacks every day. This proactive practice supports you in avoiding away from last-minute choices, which typically lead to less healthy alternatives. When your supper plan is set up, establish a grocery list. Take a look at your storage space and an ice chest to identify the things you now have and jot down what you desire to get. Having a far-reaching buying list smoothes out your purchasing for food and forestalls needless purchases. Besides, it ensures that you have every one of the fixings you require to execute your feast prep plan.

Concerning feast planning, consider entrees that may be group-made and simply split. Broiling a huge platter of veggies, preparing a major clump of complete grains like quinoa or earthy-colored rice, and putting up a protein supply (like grilled chicken or prepared tofu) may be the basis of a few meals over time. Having these pieces fully established lets you mix and combine to construct shifting and altered feasts. Put resources into superior capacity partitions to separate your pre-arranged meals. Clear holders make it uncomplicated to observe what's within, and distributing quite a deal early forestalls indulging. Separate meals into different pieces or parts so you may swiftly gather a fair plate when you're set to eat.

Name your pre-arranged feasts with the date they were produced to assure you're devouring them when they're still fresh. While several cooked dinners may stay in the ice chest for a couple of days, consider freezing any feasts you will not be enjoying within that period. This jams their quality and forestalls food waste. Recall that assortment is key to maintaining up with your energy for supper prep. While you may set up a couple of fundamental feasts, try to include numerous cuisines, culinary methods, and surfaces to make things exciting. This forestalls boredom and motivates you to anticipate your prepared supper.

Integrate some culinary tricks to speed up the meal prep process. For instance, employing a slow cooker or Moment Pot might save expenses. Pre-slashing fixings, similar to onions, garlic, and peppers, might also substantially reduce planning time.

Day 14: Careful Extravagance: Getting a charge out of Treats Virtuous

Careful excess is a technique that drives you to savor sweets and appreciate them without responsibility. A fair technique appreciates the satisfaction of indulging in your #1 food source while retaining a strong connection with eating. By utilizing mindful extravagance, you may enjoy delights that meet your preferences and consider your body's needs.

Culpability and restrictive thinking surrounding liberal food variety usually lead to a tendency of overconsumption and melancholy moods. Careful guilty pleasure reverses this pattern by establishing a nonjudgmental approach toward goodies. Rather than identifying individual food sources as "awful" or "illegal," you approach them with inquiry and admiration. This adjustment in perspective helps you to engage in your goodies without feeling like you've "cheated" on your eating

One of the important aspects of cautious guilty pleasure is awareness. Give attentive attention to your body's indicators and sensations. Inquire as to whether you're eating out of certifiable hunger or then again on the off chance that it's a response to worry, fatigue, or other sentiments. If you notice that you're eating thoughtlessly, halt for a minute to assess your feelings and if you're famished. This attentiveness supports you with distinguishing between close-to-home eating and the certifiable joy in a treat.

While savoring attentively, dial back and savor each bite. Connect with your faculties - notice the surface, smell, and sort of the food. Take more modest bites and bite gently. This boosts your eating experience as well as allows your cerebrum time to enroll contentment, lowering the chance of indulging. Segment control is one more important component of mindful guilty pleasure. Rather than recklessly gobbling up a big chunk, serve yourself a more modest quantity. Along these lines, you may delight in the treat without feeling uncomfortably fat or blameworthy afterward. Assuming you require more, you normally have another tiny portion later on the off chance that you're as yet famished. Careful extravagance furthermore requires being accessible at the moment. Stay away from conducting several jobs when eating - put disruptions like cellphones, PCs, or TVs. All things considered, generates a tranquil atmosphere that enables you to focus on the meal before you. This boosts your contentment as well as aids you with sensing when you're satisfied.

It's vital to take notice that mindful guilty enjoyment doesn't imply reveling continually. Rather, it challenges you to consciously choose your sweets. If you would join in an extravagance, make it something you appreciate and savor, as opposed to consenting to something effectively accessible. This strategy aids you with establishing a sensation of satisfaction and forestalls unthinking eating.

Eventually, the purpose of careful extravagance is to establish a pleasant connection with food. By viewing sweets as a wellspring of delight as opposed to compulsion, you might postpone the sense of difficulty that usually prompts pigging out. Careful extravagance allows you to settle on cognizant selections that line up with your desires and nutritional demands, without capitulating to the bad pattern of overindulgence and responsibility.

Week 3: Fortifying Body and Brain

Reinforcing the body and brain is a complete approach to cope with upgrades in general prosperity. It comprises increasing both physical and mental flexibility via a combination of strong practices, propensities, and exercises. By zeroing in on these perspectives, individuals might discover work on genuine health, improved cerebral capabilities, and more prominent close-to-home harmony.

Actual strength is important to a sound body. Taking part in regular workout programs that consolidate cardiovascular, strength preparation, and adaptability actions might prompt expanded bulk, bone thickness, and persistence. Active work kicks off the arrival of endorphins, increasing a happy frame of mind and lowering symptoms of anxiousness. Besides, a reasonable and supplement-rich eating regimen supplies the essential fuel to bodily operations, supporting muscular growth, cerebral aptitude, and by and large imperativeness. Mental strength is also vital. Rehearses like serious contemplation, thorough breathing, and suitable rest contribute to mental clarity and close-to-home adaptability. Taking part in workouts that test the brain, like riddles, perusing, or acquiring another expertise, aids in preserving mental capabilities and may reduce the hazard of mental degeneration as one age. Fostering a growth attitude — accepting setbacks and errors as any open opportunities for learning — develops adaptability and an inspiring viewpoint.

The body and brain are intertwined, and their flourishing typically stays tightly tied. Standard exercise has been associated with working on emotional well-being, as it promotes the cerebrum's construction of synapses like serotonin and dopamine, which assume a vital role in the state of mind and inspiration. Essentially, rehearsing pressure reduction approaches works on mental clearness as well as directs cortisol levels, promoting genuine well-being.

Building key areas of strength for an organization of loved ones provides close-to-home nourishment and promotes flexibility through challenging situations. Participating in pleasant workouts and developing good relationships may promote mental prosperity and offer a sensation of having a place. Strengthening the body and brain involves a diversified technique that combines real health, mental prosperity, and social connection. Adjusting exercise, nourishment, mental practices, and social communications contributes to an amicable and pleasant existence. By investing time in both physical and mental taking care of oneself, individuals might meet extended vitality, lowered pressure, further developed core, and generally increased personal contentment.

Day 15: Natural Development: Tracking down Delight in Exercise

Natural development, generally referred to as tracking down joy in working out, is an amazing approach that concentrates on pleasure and prosperity above unbending health goals. It pushes individuals to pay attention to their bodies, accept their normal inclinations, and take part in proactive acts that offer them joy and satisfaction. This training is a breakaway from the normal vision of activity merely as a required evil, rather applauding improvement as a wellspring of enjoyment and strengthening.

In a culture typically centered on reaching clear real criteria, natural growth stands out by creating a more definite interaction with work out. As opposed to confining themselves to merciless regimens that might promote burnout, folks are recommended to study workouts that affect them. This might entail moving, climbing, swimming, playing a game, or in any case, walking in nature. The accentuation switches from calculating calories eaten or evaluating progress in pounds lifted to realizing how growth impacts one, both intellectually and honestly. Instinctive development enhances mindfulness by helping individuals to listen to their bodies' suggestions. It's linked together with understanding the distinction between real anxiety which signifies development and which suggests potential harm. This increased awareness lets individuals adjust their workouts, pace, and power in methods that concentrate on their prosperity.

Vitally, natural growth likewise divides the barrier between "exercise" and "tomfoolery." When development is at this time not a task, persons are obligated to dependably engage in it. This controlled way leads worked on emotional well-being, expanded vitality, and a more remarkable sensation of imperativeness. The opportunity to select exercises given individual inclination promotes a favorable association with one's body, enhancing body recognition and self-worth. Natural growth links up with the care development, stressing being available at the moment. This presence increases the brain-body relationship, letting folks savor the genuine vibes of growth. This might induce lowered pressure and anxiousness as well as an improved ability to cope with sentiments. Social support is an important aspect of natural growth. Partaking in development-located activities with companions or networks may create a sensation of connection and brotherhood. Sharing experiences and consolation contributes to a positive input loop, building up the joy and satisfaction gained from growth.

Instinctual growth understands that everybody's body is unusual, and there is nobody size-fits-all approach to dealing with health. By creating a thoughtful technique to cope with growth and releasing exterior pressures, individuals may track down joy and satisfaction in being active. This strategy is a wonderful advantage for breaking free from bad associations with practice and reframing the narrative surrounding growth as an outflow of taking care of oneself and self-esteem. Natural growth hails the inborn joy of being moving and welcomes the whole variety of proactive duties that revitalize satisfaction and essentialness.

Day 16: Cardiovascular Wellbeing: Lifting Your Pulse

Cardiovascular well-being is a cornerstone of by and large prosperity, and hoisting your pulse via a regular real job is a crucial technique for supporting and keeping up with it. The cardiovascular framework includes the heart, veins, and blood, operating as one to transport oxygen and supplements all through the body. Taking part in workouts that elevate pulse develops regions of strength for an efficient cardiovascular framework, prompting different medicinal benefits.

One of the primary advantages of elevating your pulse is further enhanced cardiac capacity. At the point when you take part in cardiovascular exercises, like jogging, cycling, or swimming, your heart siphons extra blood with each beat. Over the long term, this strengthens the heart muscle, making it more effective at siphoning blood all through the body. A more grounded heart may siphon more blood with less effort, bringing in a lower resting pulse and further developed flow. Raised pulse likewise increases lung limit. During cardiovascular exertion, your breathing rate rises to provide your muscles with oxygen. This extends lung limits and focuses on respiratory production. Further increased lung capacity lets the body swap oxygen for carbon dioxide, promoting greater generally speaking oxygenation of tissues effectively. Keeping a steady weight is one additional prominent benefit of cardiovascular exercise. Taking part in activities that raise your pulse burns calories, which may assist in weight reduction or weight maintenance. Customary movement, when joined with a decent eating routine, contributes to a sound body synthesis, lessening the danger of stoutness connected to medical conditions like diabetes, hypertension, and cardiovascular infection.

Cardiovascular exercise assumes a significant job in lessening the danger of coronary disease. It aids decrease with blooding strain and cholesterol levels, the two of which are key hazard variables for cardiovascular ailment.

Moreover, by advancing a sound weight and further boosting general heart capacity, cardiovascular exercise contributes to the counteraction of heart-related difficulties. Raising your pulse greatly influences emotional well-being. Taking part in ordinary cardiovascular exercise kicks off the arrival of endorphins, commonly referred to as "happy-go-lucky" chemicals. These synthetic chemicals advance a good frame of mind, reduce strain and anxiety, and enhance generally close-to-home prosperity. Many people believe that cardiovascular exercise produces a sensation of clarity and relaxation, aiding with lessening the pressures of day-to-day existence.

To effectively boost your pulse, hold back nothing 150 minutes of moderate-power high-impact exercise or 75 minutes of unbelievable force oxygen-consuming activity each week, as indicated by wellness organizations. This might be performed using diverse actions, including lively strolling, jogging, moving, or participation in group health programs. It's vital to take notice of that previous to commencing another work-out daily routine, specifically presuming you have an existing medical problem, counseling a medical services expert is sensible. They may supply customized guidance and ensure that your selected activities match up with your solitary wellness goals and prerequisites.

Day 17: Developing Fortitude: Obstruction Preparing Advantages

Developing fortitude via obstructed preparation is a powerful and amazing approach that gives numerous benefits for genuine well-being, utilitarian ability, and in general prosperity. Opposition preparation usually referred to as weightlifting or strength preparation, comprises neutralizing a power to improve muscular fortitude, tenacity, and power. Whether you're a newbie or a thoroughly prepared health devotee, adding opposition prepping into your regimen might have substantial effects.

One of the fundamental benefits of opposition preparation is the growth in weight and strength. At the point When you push your muscles with opposition, they adapt by growing and more grounded after some time. This increased muscular power works on your real look as well as supports regular activities, for example, lifting, conveying, and moving objects sans sweat. Obstruction preparation assumes a crucial role in sustaining a sturdy body structure. Muscle tissue is metabolically active, meaning it uses more calories extremely still compared with fat tissue. As you create muscle via obstacle preparation, your resting metabolic rate expands, which may aid with weight execution and the avoidance of weight gain. Furthermore, muscular development contributes to a conditioned and sculpted build.

Past manner, opposing prepping is vital for bone health. Weight-bearing actions stimulate bone growth and help with keeping up with bone thickness, lowering the chance of osteoporosis and splitting your age. This is especially crucial for females, who are more vulnerable to bone-related disorders when they go through menopause. Opposition prepping likewise supports joint wellness and reduces the chance of harm. Reinforcing the muscles surrounding joints soothes them and gives greater aid. This can be notably beneficial for individuals with joint situations like joint inflammation since it lightens anguish and further enhances portability. Taking part in opposition preparation strongly impacts general practical capability. It enhances your ability to execute day-to-day duties with more noticeable effectiveness and less effort. From climbing stairs to carrying meals, the increased muscular power and endurance gained via opposition preparation cause these activities to feel less burdening.

Besides, obstacle prepping leads to increased sports execution. Competitors usually incorporate strength preparation to improve their power, speed, and preparedness. This may translate into greater execution in various games and proactive duties. Obstruction preparation isn't merely about real advances; it moreover gives mental and close-to-home benefits. As you complete your solidarity aims and see development, you'll experience a rise in boldness and a sensation of success. The dedication and commitment necessary for dependable preparation might influence many daily concerns.

It's vital to take notice that blockage preparation might be changed to distinct health degrees. Novices might begin with bodyweight exercises or minor obstacles, steadily progressing when they become more comfortable. Legitimate structure and technique are vital to prevent wounds, so searching for advice from wellness specialists or exercise coaches may be remarkably valuable, specifically when starting. Integrating blockage prepping with your well-being regimen doesn't certainly signify going through hours at the fitness center. Short and concentrated sessions may bring tremendous rewards. Whether you use freeloads, opposition groups, or machines, the essential is constancy and mild over-burden – bit by little increasing the weight or blockage as your solidarity goes along.

Day 18: Adaptability and Equilibrium: Yoga and Extending

Adaptability and balance are important aspects of generally speaking prosperity and real health. Integrating rehearses like yoga and extending into one's regular may substantially contribute to enhancing these perspectives.

Yoga, an antique job commencing from India, has obtained giant ubiquity generally because of its complete technique to deal with well-being. One of its central requirements is increasing adaptability and balance via different postures and groups. The usual act of yoga continually increases joint versatility and muscle flexibility, bringing about higher adaptation. Postures, for example, Descending Canine, Triangle Posture, and Cobra Posture revolve around extending and stretching muscles, which improves adaptability as well as assists in lessening strain and tension. Yoga places significant regions of strength for balance. Adjusting presentations like Tree Posture, Hero III, and Hawk Posture involves focus and soundness, in this way improving both bodily and mental equilibrium. As individuals work on these postures, they create a more prominent awareness of their body's arrangement, which thusly works on generally speaking stance and coordination.

Extending, whether incorporated as a solitary action or as a portion of a workout routine daily practice, also assumes an essential job in keeping up with adaptability and balance. Dynamic stretches, which feature controlled advances via a scope of movement, aid with expanding the bloodstream and setting up the muscles for real jobs. Static stretches, then again, are beneficial for increasing adaptability by remaining firm on a footing that extends a muscle bunch for a protracted duration. Customary stretching after workouts forestalls muscular snugness and helps recovery.

Adaptability and equilibrium are related. At the point when muscles and joints are adaptable, they consider a more expanded scope of movement, making it simpler to achieve and stay up with equilibrium. Alternately, increased balance assists with forestalling wounds amid advances that threaten solidness. Both yoga and extension contribute to this harmonic interaction by improving muscular evenness, which is vital for perfect execution and forestalling wounds.

It's crucial to take notice that flexibility and adaptation don't merely apply to the real domain. These notions likewise reach out to mental and close-to-home prosperity. Participating in exercises that boost real adaptability might metaphorically change into mental adaptability - the capacity to adjust to changing situations and points of view. Essentially, achieving balance in one's life requires managing numerous perspectives, like work, relationships, and individual time generating an agreeable presence. Working yoga and stretching into a normal routine doesn't necessitate extensive spans of duty. Indeed, simply a few seconds of cautious stretching or a brief yoga meeting may give advantages. Consistency is vital; after some time, the combined influence of these procedures prompts checked enhancements in adaptability and balance.

Day 19: Mid-Week Contemplation: Quieting the Psyche

Mid-week reflection fills in as a beneficial tool to calm the brain, revitalize the spirit, and investigate the issues of a frenetic week. As the pressures of work, commitments, and day-to-day living build, pausing in contemplation may offer a sensation of calm and mental clarity that helps through to the conclusion of the week.

Contemplation, at its heart, is the act of zeroing in the brain on the present second. This training may take numerous forms, such as caring contemplation, cherishing consideration reflection, or guided representation. Mid-week reflection, particularly, gives a chance to stir things up about the town button and search for comfort in the middle of the buzzing around. During contemplation, the brain switches from its continuing manner of constant concerns and pressures to a state of present. This change isn't linked up with disposing of contemplations by and large however rather identifying them without judgment and lovingly coming back to the selected point of attention, which may be the breath, a mantra, or substantial sensations. This psychological discipline continually promotes a calmer brain and a more remarkable skill to control pressures.

Integrating mid-week reflection into a pattern brings a few benefits. It, most significantly, allows for alleviating pressure and anxiety. As the week progresses, pressure could gather, and finding a chance to reflect helps relieve this tension, bringing about a more peaceful temperament. Besides, mindfulness increases mental clarity. It enables individuals to draw back from the hubbub of interruptions and engage with their interior selves. This psychological clarity might stimulate improved autonomous direction and an extra peaceful point of view on issues. Mid-week pondering supports substantial affluence. It aids in identifying and managing sentiments, which with canning is particularly crucial during seasons of pressure. As the psych becomes out to be more sensitive to sensitivity through thought, individuals obtain a more thorough perception of their sentiments and may respond to them in a logical and estimated approach. Physiologically, contemplation sets off the unwinding response, prompting a reduction in pulse, circulatory strain, and the development of stress hormones. This genuine relaxation isn't just repairing however it addition aids generally speaking cardiovascular wellness. Via cutting off a space for mid-week contemplation, individuals successfully improve their prosperity and wellness.

Integrating mid-week contemplation doesn't involve sophisticated plans or extensive time commitments. In any instance, dedicating merely 10-15 minutes to thought may offer major rewards. Tracking down a calm and pleasing environment, emancipated from distractions, is vital. Many folks chose to ponder in the initial part of the day to build an encouraging vibe for the afternoon or at night to relax before bed.

Day 20: Mental Lift: Cerebrum Preparing and Mental Excitement

Chasing after boosting mental aptitude and improving smartness, cerebrum preparation, and mental feeling have surfaced as astounding assets. The concept of preparing the cerebrum, similar to preparing the body, is centered on the guideline of brain adaptability - the mind's capacity to revamp and adjust in light of experiences and workouts. By taking part in exercises that challenge and invigorate the psyche, folks might acquire a huge group of advantages that contribute to mental lift and generally speaking cerebrum wellness.

Cerebrum preparation incorporates a scope of workouts intended to further increase mental skills, for example, remembering, consideration, critical thinking, and handling speed. These exercises may take many shapes, from puzzles and games to online stages especially meant to evaluate mental talents. Luminosity, Lift, and CogniFit are examples of stages that give intuitive tasks to increase mental capacities.

One of the essential advantages of mind prepping is further strengthening explicit mental abilities potential. For example, memory games may increase the cerebrum's ability to review facts, while consideration-oriented workouts boost the capability to support center and disregard disruptions. Standard dedication to these efforts may prompt visible advantages in these chosen places over the long haul.

Past the rapid benefits, cerebrum preparation might potentially develop a mental hold. Mental preservation refers to the cerebrum's ability to adapt and perform truly even after age-related alterations or mental traumas. Taking part in intellectually animating exercises during life, including cerebrum preparation, is recognized to build this mental hold, conceivably postponing the beginning of mental degradation or neurodegenerative illnesses. It's vital to take notice that although mind preparation might give benefits, how much it prompts widespread mental improvement is as yet an issue of logical dispute. A few exams have shown encouraging benefits, however, others indicate that upgrades may be constrained to the specific duties provided and may not tally up to other mental skills. The sufficiency of mind preparation might likewise vary given variables including the type of activity, the strength of commitment, and individual distinctions.

Mental sensation, then again, envelops a more extensive set of activities that stress the psyche and improve mental imperativeness. Perusing, learning another dialect, playing an instrument, engaging in sophisticated leisure activities, and searching after greater education are examples of mental excitation. These tasks demand continual learning, critical thinking, and the merging of new material - all of which assist in keeping the mind fresh and adaptable. The benefits of mental stimulation stretch out beyond rapid mental enhancements. Participating in deep-rooted studying and chasing after mentally fascinating workouts has been associated with a lowered chance of mental degeneration and dementia. The "put it to work, or it will quit working for you" standard commonly applies to cerebrum wellness - maintaining the brain drawn in and dynamic throughout life can safeguard mental capacity long into advanced age.

Consolidating mind preparation and mental sensation may offer a comprehensive technique to cope with mental improvement. Cerebrum preparation activities may target particular mental talents while taking part in mentally challenging exercises gives a more extended scope of rewards. Also, variety is vital - regularly trading between various sorts of mental pursuits forestalls repetitiveness and pulls in different mental talents.

Day 21: Investigating Nature: Open air Exercises for Wellbeing

Investigating nature via open-air workouts is an innovative effort that promotes real wellness as well as boosts mental, close-to-home, and otherworldly prosperity. Drawing in with the normal universe provides a reprieve from the requirements of current-day existence and delivers an all-encompassing manner to health.

Climbing, quite possibly among the most well-known open-air movements, lets folks immerse themselves in the splendor of sights while benefitting from cardiovascular exercise. Whether traversing green trails, ascending mountains, or meandering along beachfront approaches, climbing gives a variegated spectrum of interactions that take particular care of diverse well-being degrees. The cadenced growth of strolling in nature may be deliberate, enhancing caring and lowering pressure. Cycling is one additional open-air pursuit that consolidates the joy of growth with an affiliation with nature. Investigating panoramic diversions on a bike delivers terrific cardiovascular activity as well as allows folks to go to more significant lengths and witness the altering environment. Cycling increases mental clearness and may be a communal activity when delighted with companions or relatives.

For those searching for a more visceral encounter with nature, putting up camp gives a one-of-a-kind opportunity to disengage from innovation and embrace effortlessness. Setting up a campsite, dining outdoors, and napping beneath the sky may substantially rejuvenate. Setting up camp promotes a re-visitation of essentials, fostering appreciation for the fundamentals and a more genuine respect for the everyday world.

Cultivating is a form of open-air activity that connects individuals with the soil on a more intimate level. Planting, expanding, and sustaining a nursery not only produces tangible rewards in that frame of mind of fresh produce or lively flowers nevertheless in addition delivers a sensation of desire and success. Cultivating has been exhibited to reduce pressure and enhance a pleasant frame of mind. Nature photography is a creative and critical approach to drawing in with the outdoors. Catching the numerous details of landscapes, vegetation, and fauna motivates individuals to closely examine their environmental components. Photography likewise supplies a path to self-articulation and innovativeness.

The benefits of outdoor workouts for health go beyond the real domain. Time spent in nature has been connected with lowered emotions of worry, further developed mindset, and increased experiences of delight. The Japanese custom of "woods washing," or Shinrin-Yoku, stresses the healing advantages of merely being in a forest atmosphere. Studies have revealed the way that exposure to nature may bring down the pulse, aid the invulnerable framework, and improve mental capacity. Besides, nature considerably impacts mental prosperity. Green places have been associated with bringing down degrees of unease and unhappiness. The variety, sounds, and surfaces of the regular environment produce a multisensory experience that soothingly impacts the mind. Investigating nature likewise cultivates a sense of closeness. Being encompassed by the perfection and intricacies of the regular environment encourages a shift in perspective from individual problems to a more extended understanding of the climate and the interdependence of every living thing.

PART 2

Week 4: The first Sustaining Your Internal Identity

Sustaining your identity is a vital technique that increases self-improvement, close-to-home prosperity, and a sensation of stability throughout daily life. In the middle of our hectic and usually stressful lives, carving out the chance to engage with and care for our internal selves may considerably improve our overall pleasure and contentment.

At its heart, preserving your internal identity comprises awareness and self-sympathy. It entails understanding your emotions, concerns, and wishes without judgment. This mindfulness enables you to figure out your inspirations, triggers, and areas for self-awareness. With this getting it, you may settle on intentional choices linked up with your traits and aims.

Rehearsing self-sympathy is equally vital. Treating oneself with a similar compassion and understanding you would provide a mate generates a nice inner trade. This internal emotionally supporting network checks pessimistic self-talk and fosters a healthier mental self-picture. At the point when you're caring for yourself, you're more prepared to cope with obstacles, misfortunes, and pressures.

Taking part in activities that strengthen your spirit is one more component of preserving your identity. These exercises may alter significantly, from investing energy in nature and rehearsing caring to searching after creative outlets or leisure pastimes you're eager about. Such workouts produce glimpses of exhilaration and contentment, encouraging you to recall the necessity of taking care of oneself. Taking care of oneself techniques extend past real prosperity and also involve mental and close-to-home wellness. Participating in introspection, thorough breathing practices, or writing may aid you with addressing your ideas and emotions. This contemplative practice enhances self-understanding and deep adaptability.

Fabricating and keeping up with meaningful connections is one additional facet of preserving your internal identity. Sound relationships contribute to your overall prosperity, bringing support, solace, and the sensation of having a home. Imparting your contemplations and experiences to believing folks provides a source for articulation and eases feelings of detachment. Defining limitations is crucial for maintaining your identity. Describing limitations in various elements of your existence, including employment, relationships, and individual leisure, forestalls burnout and ensures you disperse energy to the main thing to you. Embracing self-awareness as a continual adventure is a critical mindset when keeping your own identity. Take a swing at development instead of flawlessness, and consider setbacks as any open opportunities for learning. Commend your successes along the way, regardless of how modest they may look.

Day 22: Overseeing Pressure: Methods for Unwinding

In the current high-speed environment, monitoring strain has changed into a prerequisite for keeping up with generally speaking success. Stress may damage mental, deep, and actual well-being, making it crucial to take strong unwinding approaches. Integrating these procedures into your routine may help you with relaxing up, lower pressure, and generate a sensation of balance. Here are a few processes for unwinding that may help supervise pressure;

1. Profound Relaxing: Profound breathing practices are an easy but potent way to quiet the brain and body. By taking slow, full breaths and zeroing attention on each breathe in and breathe out, you perform the body's unwinding response. This technique may be drilled wherever making it a beneficial gadget for controlling pressure consistently

2. Moderate Muscle Unwinding: This technique usually discharges real pressure and progresses unwinding. Beginning at the toes and continuing progressively up to the head, this exercise supports you with turning out to be more receptive to your body's feelings.

3. Care Contemplation: Care reflection comprises pointing out your present second without judgment. By noting your concerns, emotions, and sensations as they come, you create distance from stresses and foster a sense of stillness. Standard care practice may boost

your ability to supervise strain in a more segregated and formed approach.

4. **Directed Symbolism:** Directed symbolism takes you on a psychological vacation to a quiet and relaxing environment. Through stunning depictions, you connect with your faculties and create a psychological departure from pressures. This process takes advantage of the psyche's capacity to affect the body's pressure response, prompting unwinding.

5. **Paying attention to Music:** Music has the potential to alter moods and produce a quiet atmosphere. Slow-beat or instrumental music might bring down pulse and circulatory tension, inspiring unwinding. Make playlists of your #1 loosening-up tracks to pay attention to during worrisome situations.

6. Nature Association: Investing energy in nature might fundamentally alleviate strain. Whether it's going for a walk in the recreation area, sitting by a waterway, or climbing in the forest, soaking yourself in regular natural components may bring a sensation of serenity and point of view.

7. Imaginative Outlets: Taking part in creative activities like works of art, creating, or playing an instrument may operate as a sort of self-articulation and stress help. These outlets supply a path to channeling sentiments and diverting the center from pressures.

8. Actual work: Ordinary action releases endorphins, which are normal state-of-mind enhancers. Participating in genuine labor, whether it's jogging, moving, or swimming, might lighten strain and work on generally speaking prosperity.

Day 23: Close to home Flexibility: Exploring Life's High highlights and negative moments

Profound flexibility is the ability to experience life's highs and lows with effortlessness and variety. An essential skill engages individuals to suffer misfortune, monitor strain, and have an uplifting outlook even with challenges. Similarly, as genuine health sustains the body's prosperity, personal flexibility fortifies the psyche and soul, letting individuals return from accidents and thrive in various situations.

The basis of close-to-home strength is the capacity to regulate one's emotions. This means acknowledging and accepting emotions without judgment and later hunting out good methods of dealing and expressing them. As opposed to stifling or repressing feelings, truly strong individuals challenge them head-on, letting themselves mourn, feel the wrath, or encounter problems when required. This capacity to draw in with sentiments makes it ready for significant healing and growth. By staying present at the moment, individuals may more quickly cope with their reactions to stress. Care rehearses like contemplation and deep breathing contemplate a wait between improvement and reaction, offering the chance to decide on a clever response over an instinctive one. This skill is particularly valuable during challenging times since it forestalls foolish decisions motivated by elevated sentiments.

One foundation of deep flexibility is retaining areas of strength for a company. Interfacing with companions, relatives, or care groups gives a sense of having a home and reminds folks that they're in good company in their fights. These connections give both close-to-home approbation and down-to-earth aid when necessary, going about as a buffer against the unfavorable results of tension and misfortune. Positive self-talk is an indication of close-to-home flexibility. People who have this characteristic substitute gloomy and self-decisive contemplations with reasonable and facilitating ones. This inner discourse forms an image of obstacles, permitting them to be considered as any open doors for improvement as opposed to illusory deterrents. By reexamining conditions, individuals preserve a confident point of view that propels their adaptability. Adaptability is an important components of experiencing life's flighty twists. Sincerely tough individuals perceive change as a chance for new contacts and learning. They embrace changes with a receptive attitude, comprehending that even despite the discomfort, there's room for self-improvement and broader vision.

Developing a sense of direction helps to close to home strength. At the point when individuals have a fair understanding of their characteristics and ambitions, they're more prepared to track down relevance in obstacles. This sensation of direction goes about as a primary incentive throughout tough periods, guiding decisions and offering energy to press on. It's crucial to take notice that deep flexibility doesn't imply avoiding away from gloomy sentiments or unpleasant moments out and out. All things being equal, constructing an institution sustains substantial prosperity, helping individuals to endure hardship and stresses while preserving a sense of equilibrium. Creating close-to-home flexibility is a long-term expedition that involves attention, practice, and a willingness to ask for support when necessary.

Day 24: Appreciation and Energy: Moving Your Viewpoint

Appreciation and vitality are two great qualities that may entirely alter our lives by shifting our point of view. On a planet usually loaded with obstacles and weaknesses, accepting these traits might prompt better prosperity and a really pleasant presence. Appreciation is the act of noticing and appreciating the good elements of our existence. It entails recognizing the endowments, of all shapes and sizes, that we usually underestimate. By increasing appreciation, we teach our psyches to fix in on excess as opposed to lack. This shift in context may induce extended pleasure and happiness.

The logical study has demonstrated that repeating thankfulness consistently may bring about an improved mindset, greater slumber, and, surprise, lessened symptoms of anxiousness. At the point that we actively halt to ponder the items we're thankful for, we build a positive criticism circle that improves our general point of view. Inspiration enhances appreciation by influencing the method in which we understand circumstances and interactions. An inspiring attitude doesn't entail overlooking obstacles or challenges; rather, it means pushing toward them with a mindset of power and progress. By reframing problems as any open doorways for learning and self-improvement, we can defeat snags all the more genuinely. Energy doesn't prevent the presence from having negative sentiments; all things being equal, it motivates us to cope with them firmly and discover silver linings even in predicaments.

Moving one's perspective toward appreciation and inspiration involves deliberate labor and practice. One effective technique is maintaining an appreciation journal. Routinely jotting down things we're thankful for helps foster a happy outlook. Furthermore, zeroing in on the present second via caring routines may aid us with entirely recognizing life's uncomplicated delights. Taking part in thoughtful acts and giving thanks to others likewise cultivates a sense of connectivity and builds up nice feelings. Encircling oneself with good influences, whether via connections or media usage, may be an optimistic perspective taking part in exercises that deliver a, and chasing after hobbies may also lift one's general impression of vitality.

Over the long term, these routines become continual, little by bit rewriting the cerebrum to default to an inspired viewpoint.

It's vital to take notice that embracing admiration and inspiration doesn't imply dismissing the problems or gloomy thoughts that occur. It's linked up with hunting down a harmony between acknowledging the trials and resolving to hone in on the upsides. This harmony helps us to experience life's high moments and low points with power and effortlessness.

Day 25: Taking care of oneself Customs: Spoiling Your Body and Soul

Taking care of oneself habits assumes a critical function in supporting both the body and the soul, supplying a break from the requirements of day-to-day existence and advancing general prosperity. These rituals concentrated on spoiling and maintaining, enabling individuals to re-energize and reconnect with themselves more fundamentally.

Actual taking care of oneself is crucial for keeping up with fantastic health and essentialness. Spoiling the body with rituals like loosening up showers, skin care programs, and back massages enhances relaxing as well as encourages a pleasant self-perception, and elevates confidence. Taking part in typical exercise, whether it's yoga, jogging, or moving, retains the body healthy as well as supplies endorphins that enhance the temperament. Focusing on good nourishment, keeping hydrated, and ensuring suitable rest is fundamental to taking care of oneself in routines that support the body's genuine advancement. Past the physical, taking care of oneself reaches out to nurturing the soul and close-to-home success. Care and contemplation are rehearsed that let folks build mindfulness, lessen strain, and produce mental clearness. Participating in leisure activities and workouts that offer joy and satisfaction helps to a sense of direction and fulfillment. Setting apart some space to peruse, create, paint, or take part in other creative pastimes may be staggeringly restorative.

Investing energy in nature is one more great way to concentrate on the spirit. Whether it's a nice walk in the park or an end-of-the-week retreat to the mountains, interacting with the regular environment has been exhibited to reduce strain and work on by and large psychological well-being. Being in nature helps care and aids individuals with obtaining a point of view on life's issues. Defining good boundaries and finding out how to say "no" when necessary is equally a crucial aspect of taking care of oneself. This involves remembering one's cutoff points and realizing that OK to refuse obligations or workouts that can waste energy or produce unreasonable pressure. Saying "no" conscientiously and decisively lets individuals shield their prosperity and distribute time for activities that truly match up with their characteristics and goals. Social ties are crucial to taking care of oneself too. Investing energy with friends and family, companions, and relatives provides a sensation of having a place and support. Participating in big dialogues and maintaining contacts contribute to deep prosperity and offer a place to discuss pleasures and troubles.

Integrating taking care of oneself rites into day-to-day life takes aim and accountability. Making a standard that integrates components of physical and deep contemplation might prompt persistent benefits. It's memorable's crucial that taking care of oneself isn't juvenile; it's an interest in one's wellness and delight, which thus lets folks make an appearance all the more fully in their connections and tasks. Fitting taking care of oneself traditions to individual preferences is vital. What works for one person usually won't resound with another. The goal is to try different things with varied exercises and works, concentrating on what brings the greatest joy, relaxation, and a sensation of renewal. Routinely considering and adjusting care of traditions when situations change and essential over the long haul.

Day 26: Imaginative Articulation: Tracking down Bliss in Creative Endeavors

Imaginative articulation is a substantial and enjoyable way of tracking down pleasure and fulfillment throughout daily living. Taking part in creative initiatives enables individuals to take advantage of their internal imagination, connect with their sentiments, and experience a sensation of success that gives tremendous pleasure. Whether via artistic expressions, music, composing, or various sorts of imaginative articulation, the demonstration of generating something original and important contains the impact to improve our lives in countless ways. Imaginative endeavors provide a station for self-revelation and self-articulation. Making handicrafts allows individuals to convey ideas, sentiments, and situations that may be hard to carry on via words alone. It gives a haven of sanctuary for studying contemplations and feelings, enabling a more thorough knowledge of oneself. Through the most typical manner of creating, individuals might reveal stowed-away gifts, stand up to obstacles, and grow a more remarkable identity assurance.

The exhibition of producing craftsmanship is in many instances combined with a sensation of flowing, when time seems to stop and tensions dissipate. This situation of "stream" comes when a person is entirely immersed in a creative movement and experiences a heightened sensation of focus and pleasure. Taking part in imaginative undertakings provides a break from the requirements of day-to-day existence and offers a form of contemplation that may lessen anxiety and advance unwinding. Besides, the course of creative articulation energizes trial and error and an eagerness to welcome botches. It creates an atmosphere where it isn't simply recognized and applauded for overcoming obstacles. This attitude may reach out beyond craftsmanship itself, encouraging individuals to move toward life's issues with an additional open and varied perspective. The adaptability developed by imaginative exploration might alter critical thinking capacities and augment one's capability to adjust to change. Craftsmanship has the marvelous power to link humans across civilizations and centuries. Through visual handiwork, music, writing, and various frameworks, individuals might communicate their innovative ideas and connect on a human level. Inventive articulation evolves into an all-encompassing language that rises beyond hindrances and considers the exchanging of ideas and sentiments. This sensation of attachment might provide a considerable impression of having a place and a more expanded perspective on the globe.

For others, creative articulation fills in as a supply for treatment and healing. Craftsmanship can assist individuals in coping and adjusting to problematic sentiments, injuries, and life problems. Taking part in creative activities may provide a sensation of authority over one's tale and suggest a direction of transformation and progress. Composing, painting, and many sorts of articulation allow individuals to give voice to their experiences, bringing a sensation of closure and strengthening.

Creative ventures likewise urge an enthusiastic approach to dealing with existence. The display of creating is many times connected by a sensation of fascination and amazement, similar to how children study their general environment. This honest spirit invites individuals to embrace their creative minds, break loose from routine, and strive toward existence with a sense of peculiarity and zeal. Integrating imaginative articulation into day-to-day existence doesn't necessitate proficient preparation or uncommon talent. What makes the most difference is the demonstration of drawing in with the cycle, not the finished output. Whether it's yingling staring, playing the guitar, or writing down contemplations in a journal, carving out the opportunities for inventive activities might stimulate a more pleasant and meaningful existence.

Day 27: Computerized Detox: Adjusting Screen Time

In the modern closely associated world, the notion of a "computerized detox" has received popularity. As we grow more reliant on our screens for work, communication, enjoyment, and data, the need to modify our screen time and withdraw from the virtual realm has become more crucial than at any time in recent memory.

A digital detox comprises consciously and momentarily disengaging from modern electronics including mobile phones, tablets, PCs, and even smartwatches. The purpose is to recover a sensation of care, re-energize our psychological and real prosperity, and rebuild vital relationships with the unconnected globe. The rising of screen-based activities has caused questions regarding the possible harmful implications on our psychological well-being, connections, and generally speaking personal contentment. Inordinate screen usage has been associated with difficulties, for example, computerized eye strain, disturbed rest designs, expanded sensations of tension, and a lessened ability to focus. Subsequently, including a computerized detox into our routines may work as a counterbalance to these effects.

One of the major benefits of a computerized detox is the possibility to engage in activities that foster inventiveness and take care of oneself. Turning off screens drives us to explore leisure pastimes like artwork, producing, perusing genuine publications, or taking part in outdoor exercises. This alteration in the center lets us be accessible at the moment and interact with our ambient factors, motivating lessened pressure and working on mental clarity. A digital detox might act on our relationship connections. With less time spent attached to devices, we have the extra possibility to engage in crucial talks and emotional interactions with loved ones. It tends to be an occasion to recover the joy of eye-to-eye conversations, bolstering securities that might have been strained by the continual presence of innovation. Carrying out a profitable computerized detox incorporates creating clear restrictions for screen use. Making specified "without tech zones" at home, such as the lounge area or room, may aid with setting out a healthier balance. Saving specified seasons of day to segregate and engage in distinct workouts, for example, during feasts or before sleep time, might equally help the cycle. Organizations and associations are furthermore discovering the importance of computerized detox for their representatives' well-being. A few companies are carrying out methods that push representatives to disconnect after work hours to forestall burnout and promote a better balance between important and pleasant activities. This boosts job satisfaction as well as urges enhanced efficiency throughout working hours.

Day 28: Social Prosperity: Cultivating People Group Associations

Social prosperity, a crucial component of generally speaking well-being, revolves around the quality and power of our connections and affiliations with others. In a moment set apart by mechanical progress and advanced associations, promoting local area associations has grown much more critical to upgrading our social prosperity.

Individuals are essentially social creatures, built to search for companionship, having a location, and a sense of local region. Solid social ties have been associated with numerous physical, mental, and close-to-home benefits. They contribute to bringing down sensations of tension, working on resistive capacity, expanding confidence, and a more significant sense of contentment. Creating and nurturing these relationships is crucial for a healthy and fulfilled existence.

One technique for expanding local area associations is by effectively taking part in neighborhood events and gathers. Taking part in activities like local area cleanups, studios, good cause events, or nearby games groups not only lets people reward their areas in addition works with the creation of substantial affiliations with similar individuals. Such provides common division cooperation and shared encounters, enhancing the security within the local region. Besides, chipping in is a solid way to build relationships while having a favorable effect. Chipping in benefits the recipients of the help as well as the real employees. It delivers a sensation of purpose, enables folks to contribute to issues they are ardent about, and introduces them to new opinions. Through chipping in, folks might create relationships with others from diverse backgrounds, broadening their communities of friends and better understanding how they could view the world. Making and preserving substantial areas of strength for an ethical area likewise fundamentally assists social prosperity. Neighbors who know and support each other might generate more secure and more lively situations. Online people groups focused on common interests supply roadways to associate in any case, when genuine proximity isn't viable. These computerized networks may be particularly beneficial for persons with specialized side interests or those searching for aid and understanding from others who have comparable situations.

In the working environment, growing local area associations might stimulate greater job contentment and further expand coordinated effort. Organizations that encourage group-building activities, open communication, and a sense of fellowship among representatives will usually grow a nicer workplace. At the point when individuals sense a sensation of having a place at work, their general prosperity is affected, prompting expanded efficiency and lessened turnover.

Schooling likewise assumes a crucial function in creating local area connections. Schools and colleges that stress collaboration, group initiatives, and extracurricular activities provide open doors to understudies to key areas of strength and nurturing relationships that typically persist beyond their scholastic years. These associations may be a major wellspring of support, systems administration, and self-improvement.

Week 5: Reflection and Then Some

Reflection is a powerful mental cycle that helps individuals to dig into their interactions, contemplations, and sentiments. It fills in as a psychological mirror, permitting us to obtain an understanding of our actions, choices, and inspirations. Past its surrounding beneficial aspects, introspection works with self-awareness and progress.

At its heart, reflection encompasses study and research. A planned pause permits us to review prior circumstances and their influence on our lives. Through this cycle, we may identify designs, perceive our advantages and deficiencies, and decide on further knowledgeable selections going forward. Mindfulness, a fundamental outcome of reflection, permits us to grasp our reactions, contemplations, and methods of responding in varied settings.

Reflection isn't constrained to the unique level; it's likewise necessary in aggregate circumstances. Groups and associations that support intelligent practices usually end up more prepared to adapt to change and benefit from their encounters. By thinking about the two accomplishments and disappointments, they enhance approaches, promote teamwork, and nurture progress. Past personal progress and hierarchical learning, reflection broadly influences society. It energizes compassion by letting us think about the views of others and comprehend their experiences. This may be particularly crucial in settling social concerns and fostering inclusion. Intelligent individuals are obliged to take part in big talks, bridge gaps, and contribute strongly to their networks. Be that as it may, reflection may likewise be demanding. It demands a preparedness to face up to difficult discoveries, detect botches, and confront errors. It requires time and mental effort, which may be daunting in a fast-paced environment. In a swiftly expanding mechanical setting, fostering contemplation confronts new problems. The continual bombardment of data, interruptions, and the effort to stay "connected" might disturb our ability to genuinely contemplate. Adjusting the benefits of innovation with the need for contemplation is a precarious errand.

To revitalize appearance in our lives, we might take on numerous approaches. Journaling, pondering, and care rehearses provide committed areas to thinking. Consistently creating a chance for pondering and asking for feedback from believed persons may boost the intelligence cycle. Introspection is an everlasting habit of modern importance. It enables us to journey into our history, figure out our present, and envisage our future. By embracing introspection, we encourage self-improvement as well as contribute decisively to our relationships, working settings, and societal orders. It's a signal leading us beyond the surface layer of our contacts, into a more fundamental awareness of ourselves and our broader environment.

Day 29: Observing Advancement: Recognizing Your Accomplishments

Celebrating progress is an important aspect of self-awareness and motivation. Recognizing your triumphs, regardless of how minor they can seem, contributes to a good viewpoint and impels you along on your journey toward your goals. Perceiving and enjoying progress increases your confidence as well as fills in as an indication of your capabilities and the distance you've gone.

Frequently, folks fixate on the end target and neglect the gradual progress that takes them there. Notwithstanding, advancement is a series of tiny victories that prepare for improvement. Commending these successes offers sanction to your attempts and strengthens your responsibility for your ambitions.

Recognizing successes fosters a sense of achievement. It's a technique of giving yourself credit for the rigorous effort, devotion, and consistency you've displayed. This affirmation doesn't need to be enormous; simply a plain gesture of congrats or a picture of self-commendation may capably improve your self-esteem and assurance.

Celebrating accomplishments likewise assumes an important role in keeping up with force. At the moment when you discover a chance to appreciate what you've done, you build a positive input circle. The pride fills your inspiration, motivating you to keep pursuing your aims with renewed drive. This encouraging input might forestall fatigue and offer a sensation of direction in your activities.

Moreover, recognizing progress aids you in observing your growth and improvement. Frequently, self-improvement is gradual and may not be instantly evident. By frequently noticing and commending your efforts, you're ready to realize the considerable progress you've achieved after some time. This attention may be particularly motivating during instances when you might feel stale or hindered. Notwithstanding private benefits, commending advancement might affect those around you. Your wins might motivate others to chase after their aims and celebrate their accomplishments. Sharing your travels and applauding successes may generate a constant and empowering atmosphere that supports collective growth and vitality.

To properly celebrate progress, it's vital to set forward fair targets and identify what makes an achievement. This might range from concluding a venture at work to attaining a health objective or earning progress in an individual side interest. Separating your larger goals into more little, reasonable advancements not only makes the development path less overwhelming in addition provides more open doors to celebration along the route. Festivities may take numerous forms, depending upon your preferences and the purpose of the achievement. They might be pampering oneself with something particularly fantastic, transferring your wealth to friends and family, or basically stopping for a minute of meditation to honor your achievements.

Day 30: Supporting Genuine Wellbeing: Your Continuous Excursion

Supporting real well-being is a constant adventure that contains a complete strategy to deal with success. Genuine wellness reaches out to the basic absence of sickness; it involves physical, mental, and close-to-home components of your existence. This adventure takes unremitting effort, concentration, and a promise to pursue beneficial selections that improve your overall wellness.

At the basis of fostering true well-being is the notion of homeostasis. Adjusting real job, nourishment, relaxation, and stress the board contributes to a strong beginning point for profitability. Customary exercise increases cardiovascular wellness and strength as well as supplies endorphins that encourage mindset and mental clarity. Focusing on a reasonable and supplement-rich eating regimen supplies the essential structural obstructs your body needs to optimally operate. Also, decent slumber is vital for genuine recuperation, cerebral aptitude, and deep adaptability. Viable pressure the executive's treatments, like contemplation or care, are crucial for forestalling the hampering repercussions of persistent weight on both your body and mentality. Besides, encouraging real health needs establishing a good attitude and preserving your psychological and close-to-home success. Rehearsing self-sympathy and understanding your feelings are key to this cycle. Taking part in exercises you like, keeping up with social connections, and asking for competent aid when you want to contribute to a solid close-to-home scene. Normal well-being check-ups and screenings assume a crucial function in providing real wellness. Anticipation and early identification are crucial to reacting to possible medical issues before they become more severe. These arrangements provide an incredible opportunity to evaluate worries, obtain guidance, and adjust your wellness strategy based on the occasion.

A fundamental aspect of the continual wellness attempt is identifying realistic and attainable targets. These targets might be related to weight the board, health successes, stress reduction, or any other location of your prosperity. By breaking greater aims into more little, acceptable advancements, you may produce a sensation of success and keep up with motivation all through the excursion.

Supporting real wellness likewise incorporates staying informed and adaptable in a fast-influencing planet. The wellness scene regularly advances with fresh investigations, patterns, and innovations. Staying open to fresh facts while essentially examining legitimacy encourages you to decide on educated judgments that line up with your distinct wellness demands.

Developing areas of strength for a framework is one additional basis for your continual wellness attempt. Encircling oneself with individuals who share your commitment to welfare may offer comfort, responsibility, and a sensation local calla. Whether it's a workout friend, a nourishment group, or a web-based discussion, a strong organization may make your trip more pleasurable and supportable.

In the middle of the pursuit of true wellness, adopting taking care of oneself as a non-debatable practice is crucial. Carving aside margin for oneself, whether it's via amusement activities, relaxing, or side hobbies, is important for re-energizing and keeping up with equilibrium. Taking care of oneself isn't infantile; it's an interest in your success that ultimately benefits both you and everyone around you. As you develop on your wellness journey, difficulties are inevitable. These errors are not disappointments but rather opportunities to learn and improve. Versatility and perseverance are crucial traits in sustaining true wellness. When presented with challenges, regard them as temporary road impediments instead of unpleasant hindrances. Gain from challenges, adjust your methods and continue to push on with recharged certainty.

Exercise Manual for Living

Good Objective Setting:

Actual Real Health Objective: Exercise 3 times per week for 30 minutes

Activity Steps:

- Exploration exercise routine programs
- Arrange practice time
- Monitor progress.

Mental and Close to Home Wellbeing Objective: Practice reflection for 10 minutes every day

Activity Steps:

- Monitor down an acceptable reflection technique.
- construct a calm location.

- Monitor day-to-day practice.

Scholarly Wellbeing Objective: Read one book per month on a different subject

Activity Steps:

- Pick books.

- Establish understanding timeline.

- Make notes on main takeaways.

Social Wellbeing Objective: Interface with a companion or family each week

Activity Steps:

- Timetable calls or trips.

- connect well in chats.

Otherworldly Wellbeing Objective: Burn through 15 minutes in nature or intellectual practice every day

Activity Steps:

- Pick open-air workouts.

- Arrange a peaceful area inside.

- Analyze experiences.

Conclusion

Carrying on with a good every day extends beyond a basic daily plan; it takes persistent thinking and meaningful effort. Reflection, in this particular instance, pertains to the process of searching inside to review one's actions, behaviors, and attitude. This introspection enables individuals to tailor their lives to their traits and aspirations, generating a sense of purpose and fulfillment.

At the root of living great is the recognition that every day is an opportunity for progress. By providing time for contemplation, folks may separate locations where they excelled and aspects that demand better. This program increases awareness and raises a proactive strategy to cope with self-improvement. Through reflection, one may celebrate triumphs and acknowledge progress, promoting confidence and motivation.

Moreover, reflection helps the ID of instances and propensities, both good and negative. This awareness motivates individuals to build up useful ways to resolve ones. someone could perceive that spending an excess of energy on web-based amusement leaves them feeling tired and worthless. Outfitted with this information, people may purposefully limit screen time and divide those minutes into hobbies that elevate and develop their lives.

Notwithstanding, meditation alone isn't enough; it should be supplemented with conscious action. Making an interpretation of experiences into real changes is the cornerstone of growth. This might entail creating achievable aims that match up with specific attributes or making aware actions that improve bodily, mental, and deep success. For example, a person contemplating their sedentary propensities may concentrate on an everyday walk or workout routine daily program.

Living wonderful likewise envelops preserving relationships and collaborations. Considering cooperation with others might encourage improved communication, compassion, and understanding. Offering gratitude and appreciating the good influence of friends and family sets up relationships and enables a pleasant environment. To support these efforts, establishing timelines and frameworks is crucial. Standard reflection sessions, writing, or contemplation may become essential components of day-to-day living. Additionally, retaining a receptive attitude and responding to change considers constant progress and forestalls stagnation. As situations develop, so too should the techniques for living excellent. The expedition of continuing with normal daily living reaches well beyond superficial timetables. It comprises steady reflection when individuals examine their behaviors, values, and ambitions. Through contemplation, good propensities are built up, bad instances are responded to, and awareness is enhanced. Thinking alone isn't adequate; deliberate conduct is important to transform an interpretation of encounters into actual adjustments. This might entail putting out aims, maintaining ties, and concentrating on prosperity. By accepting these principles and keeping open to improvement, individuals may depart on a fulfilling journey of ongoing personal progress and a daily routine very fully experienced.